The journey for a healthy life:

Secrets for maintaining a healthy diet and achieving weight loss.

By

Angela Robertson

The journey for a healthy life.

**Copyright © Angela Robertson
2023. All rights reserved**

This document must first have permission from the publisher before being copied or otherwise replicated.

The journey for a healthy life.

TABLE OF CONTENT

INTRODUCTION.

Food diets are eating plans that concentrate on particular food groups or macronutrient ratios in order to enhance health, avoid disease, and control weight. Many people find it difficult to maintain a balanced diet in today's environment due to the variety of food options. Food plans provide a planned way to eat that can assist people in achieving their nutritional objectives, whether they be for illness prevention, greater athletic performance, or weight loss.

There are many different kinds of dietary diets, each with its own set of rules and limitations. While some diets, like the vegan and vegetarian diets, place a strong emphasis on avoiding animal products, others, like the ketogenic and low-carb diets, place a restriction on the amount of carbohydrates consumed. Choosing the correct eating diet might be difficult because there are so many options accessible. However, anyone may find a food regimen that fits their own needs and interests with the correct advice and information.

The journey for a healthy life.

Food diets can provide difficulties, such as navigating social situations and controlling desires for food, even though they have some advantages. However, people can successfully implement and maintain a food diet with proper planning and support. In this manual, we will examine various food plans, how to select the best one, and how to deal with typical difficulties. You will have the information and resources necessary to begin your own food diet journey and reach your dietary objectives by the end of this course.

CHAPTER 1.

DEFINITION:

A food diet is a planned eating strategy that places an emphasis on particular food groups, macronutrient ratios, or food kinds in order to enhance general health, avoid disease, or control weight. A normal food diet is making decisions about what and how much to eat in accordance with a set of rules or limitations. Personal objectives, dietary requirements, and lifestyle considerations may influence these recommendations. A diet can be short-term or long-term, and it can involve including or excluding particular foods or dietary groups. An ideal food diet supports general health and well-being by optimizing nutrient consumption.

IMPORTANCE OF FOOD DIET.

Food diets are crucial for a number of reasons, such as:

Nutritional Intake: Adhering to a food plan can help people consume a balanced, diverse diet that satisfies their nutritional requirements. This can guard against nutritional deficiency and advance general wellness.

Disease Prevention: It has been demonstrated that certain dietary diets, such the Mediterranean and DASH diets, lower the risk of chronic illnesses like cancer, diabetes, and heart disease. A diet high in fruits, vegetables, whole grains, and lean protein can supply crucial nutrients that fight disease and lower the chance of developing chronic illnesses.

Weight Control: Many dietary diets are created to encourage weight loss or weight maintenance. People can manage their weight and improve their general health by choosing foods that are high in nutrients and limiting their portion sizes.

Energy and Performance: People can get the nutrients and energy they need to support physical activity and athletic performance from a diet that is well-balanced. Protein, carbs, or healthy fats may be prioritized in specialized dietary regimens for athletes and active people.

Mental Health: According to research, certain food diets, like the Mediterranean diet, can support mental health and lower the chance of developing sadness and anxiety. The brain's health and mood can be supported by eating a diet high in omega-3 fatty acids, B vitamins, and antioxidants.

In conclusion, dietary diets are crucial for preserving general health and wellbeing. Individuals can maximize their nutritional intake, prevent disease, manage weight, and promote physical and mental performance by adhering to a diet that is customized to their requirements and goals.

BENEFITS OF MAINTAINING A HEALTHY DIET

The advantages of maintaining a healthy diet are numerous and include:

Improved Nutritional Intake: A healthy diet offers a balanced and diverse intake of nutrients that are necessary to keep one's health at its best. This can guard against vitamin deficits and advance general health.

Weight management: Eating a balanced diet reduced in added sugars, processed carbs, and saturated and trans fats can help people reach and maintain a healthy weight. This can lessen the likelihood of developing obesity and its related health issues.

Reduced chance of Chronic Diseases: Research has shown that eating a balanced diet high in fruits, vegetables, whole grains, lean protein, and healthy fats lowers the chance of developing chronic conditions including heart disease, diabetes, and some cancers.

Better Mental Health: Consuming a balanced diet full of vitamins and minerals like omega-3 fatty acids, B vitamins, and antioxidants can boost mental health and lift spirits. A nutritious diet has been found in studies to lower the chances of anxiety and depression.

Enhanced Energy and Stamina: A nutritious diet can give you the nutrition and energy you need to sustain your athletic performance. The general health and well-being can be enhanced by this.

Better Digestive Health: By encouraging regularity, decreasing constipation, and lowering the risk of digestive illnesses like diverticulitis and inflammatory bowel disease, a nutritious diet rich in fiber can enhance digestive health.

Improved Immune Function: Consuming a nutritious diet full of vitamins C, E, and zinc helps boost immunity and lower the risk of getting sick or infected.

The journey for a healthy life.

In conclusion, maintaining a balanced diet can have a variety of positive effects on your health and wellbeing in general. People can maximize their nutritional intake, lower their risk of chronic diseases, and promote both their physical and mental health by choosing a diet high in whole, nutrient-dense foods.

CHAPTER 2.

TYPES OF DIETS

VEGAN DIET.

The intake of any animal products, including meat, chicken, fish, seafood, eggs, dairy products, and honey, is prohibited on a vegan diet, which is a sort of vegetarian diet. Fruits, vegetables, legumes, grains, nuts, and seeds are the main sources of nourishment in this plant-based dietary pattern. Beyond dietary choices, veganism frequently encompasses way of life decisions that minimize harm to animals and the environment.

Benefits of a Vegan Diet for Health:

Nutritionally Sufficient: A vegan diet that is well-planned can offer all the essential elements, such as protein, carbs, healthy fats, vitamins, and minerals. Fiber, antioxidants, and phytochemicals found in plant-based diets help improve general health and lower the chance of developing chronic diseases.

Heart Health: Studies have shown a decreased risk of heart disease in people who follow vegan diets. Naturally low in saturated fat and cholesterol, plant-based diets can aid in preserving normal blood pressure and cholesterol levels.

Weight management: Compared to diets that incorporate animal products, vegan diets typically have lower calorie densities. They can therefore be a successful strategy for managing weight and lowering the risk of obesity.

Lower Risk of Chronic Diseases: Research has suggested that adopting a vegan diet may reduce your risk of getting chronic conditions like type 2 diabetes, some cancers (such colorectal cancer), and hypertension.

Improved stomach Health: Plant-based diets often contain a lot of fiber, which helps with bowel movements and encourages the growth of good bacteria in the stomach.

Environmental advantages of a vegan diet:

Reduced Greenhouse Gas Emissions: The production of animal products is a major source of greenhouse gas emissions. Individuals can lessen their carbon footprint and contribute to climate change mitigation by adopting a vegan diet.

Resources must be conserved because they are used up quickly when producing animal products on land, in water, and with energy. Changing to a vegan diet can ease the strain on ecosystems and help preserve natural resources.

Biodiversity preservation: Deforestation and habitat damage are frequent side effects of animal agriculture. Living a vegan lifestyle assists the protection of endangered animals and wildlife habitats.

Ethics: Concerns about animal welfare are frequently what drive people to become vegans. Animals should not be utilized as commodities or cruelly treated for human consumption, according to supporters of this position.

Challenges and Things to Think About:

Planning for Nutrients: While a vegan diet that is well-planned can provide nutritional requirements, specific nutrients, such as vitamin B12, iron, calcium, omega-3 fatty acids, and vitamin D, need special care. Vegans should make sure they consume these nutrients, if necessary, through fortified foods or supplements.

Social and practical considerations: Living a vegan lifestyle might be difficult when going out to eat or attending events when there aren't many vegan options available. These obstacles are, however, gradually being overcome because to rising vegan product availability, supporting communities, and more public awareness.

Personalized Approach: Individual needs and tastes can change, just like with any diet. While some people may need to make adaptations or decide to consume tiny amounts of animal products, others may flourish on a vegan diet.

The journey for a healthy life.

Before making any dietary changes, it is advised to speak with a qualified dietitian or other healthcare provider to ensure optimal nutrition and address any specific concerns.

Overall, a well-planned vegan diet can have a positive impact on the environment, improve health, and be in line with ethical principles pertaining to animal welfare.

VEGETARIAN DIET

A vegetarian diet is an eating plan that prioritizes plant-based meals while limiting or eliminating the consumption of animal products. The popularity of vegetarianism has grown over time for several reasons, including its health advantages, ethical implications, and environmental sustainability. This article will discuss several vegetarian diets, their potential advantages and drawbacks, as well as offer advice on leading a vegetarian lifestyle.

Different vegetarian diets include:

Vegetarianism that incorporates dairy products, eggs, and plant-based meals while avoiding meat, poultry, and shellfish is known as a lacto-ovo vegetarian diet.

A lacto-vegetarian diet contains dairy products and plant-based foods but forgoes seafood, poultry, and meat.

Ovo-vegetarian: A diet that consists solely of plant-based foods and eggs, with no dairy, meat, poultry, or shellfish.

Vegan: Vegans consume only plant-based foods and refrain from using any dairy, meat, poultry, seafood, eggs, or even honey.

Gains from Eating Vegetarians:

Better overall health: A vegetarian diet that is well-planned can offer all the essential elements, such as vitamins, minerals, and protein while being low in saturated fat and cholesterol. Obesity, heart disease, high blood pressure, and several cancers are often less common in vegetarians.

Increased consumption of fruits and vegetables: Vegetarians regularly eat a wide range of fruits, vegetables, whole grains, legumes, nuts, and seeds, which are packed with fiber, antioxidants, and phytochemicals. These nutrients help improve digestion, boost the immune system, and lower the chance of developing chronic diseases.

Environmental sustainability: Deforestation, water pollution, and greenhouse gas emissions are all significantly impacted by animal husbandry. Individuals can lessen their impact on the environment and support sustainable food production by switching to a vegetarian diet.

Ethics: Due to ethical worries about animal welfare and how animals are treated in the food industry, many people choose a vegetarian diet.

Dietary Considerations for Vegetarians:

Planning your nutrients: A vegetarian diet that is well-balanced can give you all the nutrients you need, but some nutrients may need extra care. These include vitamin D, calcium, iron, zinc, vitamin B12, and omega-3 fatty acids. It's crucial to make sure you're getting enough by choosing carefully which plant-based sources, taking supplements, or eating fortified meals.

Protein sources: To meet protein requirements, it's vital to eat a variety of plant-based foods, such as legumes, tofu, tempeh, seitan, quinoa, and some nuts and seeds. Throughout the day, combining various plant protein sources can help make sure that all necessary amino acids are consumed.

Meal preparation: To guarantee a balanced diet, it is essential to prepare meals in advance and include a range of plant-based foods. Making the switch to a vegetarian lifestyle fun and sustainable can be accomplished by experimenting with different dishes, flavors, and cooking methods.

Follow this Advice to Live a Vegetarian Lifestyle:

Gradual transition: To begin, gradually cut back on your intake of meat, poultry, and fish while upping your intake of plant-based foods. This strategy enables a more seamless transition and adjustment to new tastes and sensations.

Education and assistance: Gain knowledge about vegetarian nutrition, and look for assistance from vegetarian groups, internet sources, or licensed dietitians who can help you plan meals and manage any nutritional issues.

Include a wide range of fruits, vegetables, whole grains, legumes, nuts, and seeds in your meals for diversity and experimentation. To keep your diet fresh and enjoyable, explore new recipes and cuisines.

Meals that are well-balanced: Aim for meals that are well-balanced and contain a variety of carbohydrates, proteins, and healthy fats. Put bright vegetables, nutritious grains, and protein in your dish.

MEDITERRANEAN DIET

The historic eating patterns of the nations bordering the Mediterranean Sea served as the inspiration for the well-known Mediterranean diet. It has grown in popularity for its possible health advantages and has been linked to a lower risk of certain chronic diseases. The diet is renowned for its mouthwatering flavors as well as for emphasizing fresh, whole foods and a balanced diet.

Crucial Components of the Mediterranean Diet:

Fruits and vegetables in abundance: The Mediterranean diet promotes consuming a wide range of fruits and vegetables. These foods are a good source of antioxidants, fiber, vitamins, and minerals, all of which are good for general health.

Whole grains: Brown rice, whole wheat, oats, and barley are all essential components of the Mediterranean diet. They deliver fiber, complex carbs, and vital minerals.

Healthy fats are encouraged by the diet, especially the monounsaturated fats found in olive oil, avocados, and almonds. These fats increase satiety while lowering the risk of heart disease.

Lean proteins: Lean proteins included in foods like fish, fowl, lentils, and nuts are consumed in moderation in the Mediterranean diet. Fish, particularly sardines and salmon, are great providers of omega-3 fatty acids, which have been linked to several health advantages.

Red meat is taken in moderation in the Mediterranean diet, as are processed foods. Lean protein sources like fish and lentils are the main focus. Refined carbohydrates, processed meals, and sweetened beverages are also in moderation.

Spices and herbs: The Mediterranean diet relies on the use of spices and herbs to enhance the flavors of meals, lowering the need for excessive salt or added sweeteners.

There are numerous health benefits of the Mediterranean diet:

Heart disease risk is reduced thanks to the diet's concentration on heart-healthy fats like olive oil and the addition of fish as a protein source. It has been linked to lower "bad" LDL cholesterol levels and a decreased risk of heart attacks and strokes.

Weight management: Although the Mediterranean diet does not strictly adhere to calorie restrictions, it can help with healthy weight management because it places a focus on nutritious foods and sensible portion sizes. The abundance of healthy fats and high fiber content encourage fullness and prevent overeating.

Better brain health: Research suggests that eating a diet rich in fruits, vegetables, and other anti-inflammatory foods may help protect cognitive function and lower the risk of neurodegenerative disorders like Alzheimer's. These advantages may be attributed to the diet's anti-inflammatory characteristics, healthful fats, and antioxidant content.

Reduced risk of some cancers: Limiting consumption of red meat and processed meals, combined with emphasizing plant-based foods like Whole grains, fruits, and vegetables may help reduce the chance of developing certain malignancies, including colorectal and breast cancer.

Better control of diabetes: The Mediterranean diet's emphasis on whole foods, healthy fats, and complex carbs can help people with diabetes control their blood sugar levels and improve their insulin sensitivity.

It's crucial to remember that the Mediterranean diet involves a lifestyle that encourages physical activity, communal meals with family and friends, and a generally balanced attitude to eating. It's not only about the types of food that are consumed. Before making major dietary changes, it is usually important to speak with a medical practitioner or a trained dietician.

PALEO DIET

The Paleo Diet, often called the Paleolithic Diet or the Caveman Diet, is a well-liked dietary strategy that aims to resemble the dietary practices of our prehistoric predecessors from the Paleolithic era. It is predicated on the idea that meals that our hunter-gatherer predecessors ate are the ones to which the human body is most naturally adapted.

Consuming foods that would have been available to early humans during the Paleolithic period, which spanned from around 2.6 million to 10,000 years ago, is the basic tenet of the Paleo diet. This entails emphasizing whole, unprocessed foods and staying away from contemporary processed foods that were developed along with the development of agriculture.

The Paleo diet has the following essential components:

Emphasis on whole foods: The diet promotes the eating of lean meats, fish, seafood, eggs, fruits, vegetables, nuts, and seeds, as well as other fresh, unprocessed foods. These meals are said to be more nutrient-dense and more like those consumed by our ancestors.

Foods that have been processed are forbidden on the Paleo diet, including dairy products, sugar, vegetable oils, refined grains, and sugar. These foods are frequently linked to contemporary health problems like obesity, diabetes, and heart disease.

Grain and legume-free: The Paleo diet excludes grains and legumes such as wheat, rice, corn, beans, and lentils. Advocates claim that these foods can cause inflammation and digestive problems and that they were not a major component of the Paleolithic diet.

good fat sources: The Paleo diet promotes the use of good fats from foods including nuts, coconut oil, avocados, and olive oil. These fats offer both vital nutrition and energy.

Limiting added sugars: The Paleo diet forbids the consumption of added sugars including table sugar, high-fructose corn syrup, and artificial sweeteners. Instead, you can occasionally use natural sweeteners like honey or maple syrup.

The Paleo diet's proponents assert that by following this eating plan, people can lose weight, enhance their general health, and lower their risk of developing chronic diseases. It's crucial to remember that there is little scientific data to back up these claims, and researchers are still looking into the long-term impacts of diet on health.

The Paleo diet is criticized for being extremely stringent and for banning some food groups that provide vital nutrients. They also note that there is no one "Paleo" diet that correctly depicts what our predecessors ate because the Paleolithic epoch varied considerably across various geographic areas.

As with any diet, it's crucial to seek medical advice or speak with a trained nutritionist before making any major dietary adjustments. They may advise you on how to make sure you're meeting all of your nutritional needs and assist assess whether the Paleo Diet is appropriate for your particular needs.

KETOGENIC DIET

The low-carb, high-fat ketogenic diet, sometimes known as the keto diet, has become more well-known in recent years. It emphasizes cutting back on carbohydrates while upping fat consumption, which causes the body to enter a condition known as ketosis. The body predominantly uses fat for energy when it is in a state of ketosis rather than carbs.

The usual ketogenic diet calls for ingesting 70–75 percent of daily calories from fats, 25–30 percent from protein, and just 10–15 percent from carbohydrates. This macronutrient ratio encourages the generation and use of ketones, which are created by the liver when fat is broken down, to significantly reduce the body's reliance on glucose as fuel.

Changing the body's metabolism to a state of ketosis is the main objective of the ketogenic diet. Limiting carbohydrates causes the body's glycogen reserves to be depleted and lowers insulin levels. The effect is that the body begins turning lipids into fatty acids and ketones. The brain and other organs receive their energy from these ketones, which act as a substitute energy source.

The ketogenic diet's capacity to promote weight loss is one of its key advantages. By reducing carbohydrate consumption, the body is compelled to use its fat reserves as a source of energy. Significant weight loss may result from this, especially in the early phases of the diet. The diet's high fat and protein composition also aids in promoting satiety, making it simpler for people to stick to it and prevent overeating.

Additionally, it has been discovered that the ketogenic diet is beneficial for several medical issues. It has demonstrated potential for enhancing insulin sensitivity and blood sugar regulation, which is advantageous for people with type 2 diabetes or prediabetes. Although more research is required in these areas, some studies have also suggested that the ketogenic diet may have neuroprotective characteristics and could perhaps help manage illnesses including epilepsy, Alzheimer's disease, and Parkinson's disease.

The ketogenic diet has some potential advantages, but it also has some drawbacks. Initial adverse effects from the significant drop in carbohydrate intake, known as the "keto flu," can include lethargy, headaches, dizziness, and irritability. Long-term maintenance can also be challenging because it calls for careful meal planning and attention to the intake of macronutrients. In addition, the diet's high-fat content may cause people to worry about how it may affect their cardiovascular health, even though new studies indicate that the impacts on blood lipid profiles are not as dramatic as previously believed.

Before beginning a ketogenic diet, like with any diet, it is imperative to speak with a healthcare provider or certified dietitian, especially if you have any underlying medical concerns. They may offer tailored advice and guarantee that the diet is suitable for your requirements.

In conclusion, the ketogenic diet is a low-carb, high-fat eating plan that encourages ketosis and the use of fat as fuel. It has grown in popularity because of its possible advantages in terms of weight loss and specific medical issues. It may not be appropriate for everyone and requires strict adherence and monitoring to be effective.

LOW-CARB DIET.

A low-carb diet limits the consumption of carbs, which are mostly present in foods like grains, starchy vegetables, sweet meals, and some fruits. Instead, it places a focus on non-starchy veggies, healthy fats, and foods high in protein. This strategy seeks to regulate blood sugar levels, encourage weight loss, and enhance general health.

Reducing the intake of carbs, which are converted by the body into glucose and can raise blood sugar levels, is the fundamental idea underlying a low-carb diet. By restricting carbohydrates, the body is compelled to turn to fat stores for energy, which promotes weight loss.

Here are some main ideas and advantages of a low-carb diet:

Weight loss: Losing extra weight is one of the main reasons people choose a low-carb diet. By consuming fewer carbohydrates and managing insulin levels, the body is compelled to use fat reserves as energy, which leads to weight loss.

Blood sugar control: People with diabetes or insulin resistance may benefit from low-carb diets. Reducing carbohydrate intake can help control blood sugar levels, requiring less insulin and possibly enhancing insulin sensitivity.

Increased satiety: Low-carb diets are frequently linked to an increase in fullness sensations and a decrease in cravings. Foods strong in protein and good fats can make you feel fuller for longer periods, which may result in a reduction in total calorie intake.

Improved cardiovascular health: According to some studies, a low-carb diet can help with several heart disease risk factors, including lowering blood pressure, raising HDL (good) cholesterol, and reducing triglyceride levels.

greater mental focus and clarity: Some people claim that adopting a low-carb diet results in greater mental focus and clarity. While additional investigation is required to completely understand the relationship, it is thought that stable blood sugar levels and the availability of ketones as a different type of brain fuel may be important.

Better metabolic health: A low-carb diet can improve metabolic syndrome markers, lower fasting insulin levels, and reduce inflammation, all of which are indicators of better metabolic health.

It's crucial to concentrate on eating nutrient-dense foods when on a low-carb diet. Lean proteins (chicken, fish, tofu), non-starchy vegetables (broccoli, cauliflower), healthy fats (avocado, olive oil, nuts), and a small amount of low-sugar fruits should all be consumed in moderation.

It's important to remember that there is no one-size-fits-all low-carb diet. While some people might benefit greatly from a low-carb diet, others might not. It's crucial to pay attention to your body, speak with a medical expert, and tailor your strategy to your unique requirements, objectives, and health circumstances.

Finally, it's critical to sustain a balanced diet and way of life over the long run. Although a low-carb diet can help people lose weight and have some positive health effects, durability is essential. Find a long-term dietary pattern that works best for you by integrating a wide variety of nutrient-rich foods.

LOW-FAT DIET.

A low-fat diet is a dietary strategy that prioritizes cutting back on fat intake, especially trans and saturated fats. It has received a lot of attention for its possible health advantages, particularly in the treatment and management of a few chronic illnesses like diabetes, heart disease, and obesity. A low-fat diet dramatically lowers the proportion of calories from fat than a typical Western diet does.

A low-fat diet has the following important benefits:

A low-fat diet typically seeks to keep dietary fat intake between 20 and 35 percent of total daily calorie intake. As much as 35% of the calories in a typical Western diet are made up of fat, in contrast. Proteins and carbs make up the remaining calories in a low-fat diet.

Avoidable fats: In a low-fat diet, trans and saturated fats should be reduced to a minimum. Butter, full-fat dairy, fatty meats, and other animal items are common sources of saturated fats. Trans fats are fats that have been manufactured artificially and are present in many processed meals, including fried foods, baked products, and snack foods. These fats have the potential to elevate cholesterol and raise the risk of heart disease.

Sources of good fats: While a low-fat diet forbids the consumption of trans and saturated fats, it permits the consumption of good fats like monounsaturated and polyunsaturated fats. Foods like avocados, almonds, seeds, olive oil, and fatty seafood like salmon and mackerel are sources of these fats. These good fats, when consumed in moderation, can supply necessary fatty acids and other nutrients.

Dietary advantages of reduced fat:

Heart health: Limiting saturated and trans fats can help lower levels of LDL cholesterol, sometimes known as "bad" cholesterol, and lower the risk of developing heart disease and stroke.

Weight management: Since fat has a higher caloric density than proteins and carbs, a low-fat diet may be an efficient way to lose weight. When paired with a balanced diet and moderate exercise, reducing overall fat intake can help people achieve a calorie deficit and lose weight.

Diabetes management: Low-fat diets can be helpful for those with diabetes or those who are at risk of contracting the disease. Improved insulin sensitivity and blood sugar regulation may result from a diet low in saturated and trans fats.
Possible difficulties

Inadequate consumption of critical fatty acids and fat-soluble vitamins (A, D, E, and K) can cause nutrient shortages when fat intake is restricted. Nutrient-dense foods should be chosen, and if necessary, appropriate supplements should be taken into account.

Taste and satiety: Fats enhance the flavor, consistency, and satiety of meals. Finding substitute ways to improve flavors and boost enjoyment on a low-fat diet may be necessary. Some ideas include incorporating herbs, spices, and low-calorie flavorings.

The journey for a healthy life.

Sustainability: Some people may find it difficult to maintain a low-fat diet over the long term because it may call for considerable dietary changes as well as modifications to food selection and cooking techniques.

Moderating and personalizing: It's crucial to remember that a low-fat diet might not be appropriate for everyone. Dietary requirements and health objectives differ from person to person. A low-carb or Mediterranean diet, for example, maybe more advantageous for some people. To choose the best diet based on personal tastes and needs, it is essential to speak with a qualified dietitian or healthcare expert.

Keep in mind that for overall health and well-being, a balanced, diverse diet is essential, as is frequent exercise.

GLUTEN-FREE DIET.

An eating plan that doesn't include the protein gluten is known as a gluten-free diet. Grain varieties like wheat, barley, rye, and triticale frequently contain gluten. Gliadin and glutenin are two proteins that are combined to give the dough its elasticity and affect the texture of many baked items.

The main cause of people adhering to a gluten-free diet is celiac disease, a medical ailment. Gluten ingestion causes an immunological reaction that damages the small intestine and impairs nutrient absorption in those with celiac disease, an autoimmune illness. Gluten-free diets must be closely followed by those who have celiac disease to prevent symptoms and long-term problems.

The prevalence of gluten-free eating plans among people without celiac disease has grown in recent years. Due to supposed health advantages including better digestion, more energy, and weight loss, some people decide to cut gluten out of their diet. Others may develop gastrointestinal symptoms similar to those of patients with celiac disease but without the same immune response due to non-celiac gluten sensitivity.

It's crucial to carefully read product labels when adhering to a gluten-free diet because gluten can be found in unanticipated places including sauces, condiments, and processed foods. Fruits, vegetables, lean meats, fish, poultry, legumes, nuts, and dairy products are examples of naturally gluten-free foods. Rice, corn, quinoa, buckwheat, millet, and gluten-free oats are examples of grains and starches that are free of gluten. Oats, however, should be marked as gluten-free on the packaging because they are susceptible to cross-contamination with gluten during processing.

When planned properly, a gluten-free diet can be nutritious, but it's vital to remember that doing so may result in some nutritional shortages. Wheat and other whole grains that contain gluten are an important source of fiber, B vitamins, and minerals like iron and zinc. People who adopt a gluten-free diet should therefore make sure they get these nutrients from alternative sources or think about fortified gluten-free goods.

To make sure they satisfy their nutritional needs, it is advised that anyone thinking about going gluten-free without a medical reason speak with a healthcare provider or a trained dietitian. These experts may offer assistance with meal planning, assist in finding hidden sources of gluten, and offer suggestions for keeping a balanced diet.

In conclusion, those who have celiac disease or non-celiac gluten sensitivity must follow a gluten-free diet. It entails avoiding grains that contain gluten and choosing gluten-free alternatives. While adopting a gluten-free diet can be a healthy decision, it's crucial to be aware of any nutrient deficits and get medical advice before making any major dietary changes.

CHAPTER 3.

HOW TO CHOOSE THE RIGHT FOOD DIET.

The appropriate food diet is a crucial choice that can have a big impact on your health and well-being. Finding the diet trend that works for you can be difficult because there are so many of them and contradicting information is readily available. You may, however, make an informed choice regarding the best eating plan for your requirements by taking a few important elements into account and according to some general recommendations. You can follow these methods to choose the proper diet:

Establish precise objectives: Establish your goals first. Do you want to adopt a more wholesome and balanced eating pattern, reduce weight, get healthier overall, manage a particular medical condition, or all of the above? Knowing your objectives will enable you to eliminate some possibilities and select a diet that supports them.

Examine your health now: Before making any dietary adjustments, it's crucial to assess your existing state of health. Think about things like any current medical issues, dietary limitations, food allergies or intolerances, and personal preferences. A trained dietitian or healthcare expert can offer insightful advice and tailored recommendations based on your unique requirements.

Investigate several diet strategies: Learn about various diet strategies and the guiding principles behind them. Mediterranean, vegetarian or vegan, low-carb, ketogenic, paleo and intermittent fasting are a few examples of popular diets. Recognize the fundamental tenets, dietary limits or preferences, and probable advantages and disadvantages of each diet.

Think about long-term sustainability: It's important to pick a diet you can stick to in the long run. Avoid severe or excessively restrictive diets that can be difficult to follow over the long term or result in nutrient deficits. Look for a well-rounded strategy that allows for flexibility and enjoyment while including a wide range of nutrient-dense foods.

Analyze the scientific data Investigate the effectiveness and safety of a certain diet using evidence-based information. Be wary of fad diets and those that make exaggerated claims without supporting evidence. renowned sources to take into account include peer-reviewed studies, renowned health organizations, and certified dietitians' or nutritionists' expert judgments.

Observe your body: Consider how various foods make you feel. Try out different diets and track your body's reactions. Take note of any changes in your mood, digestion, level of energy, or general well-being. This self-awareness can assist you in identifying the foods that are most beneficial to you and those that you may need to limit or avoid.

Consult a professional: If you're unsure about the best diet to follow or require individualized counsel, don't hesitate to consult a qualified dietitian or nutritionist. They can evaluate your particular requirements, make recommendations that are specific to you, and help you make educated decisions regarding your nutrition.

The journey for a healthy life.

After choosing a diet, think about implementing moderate adjustments to give your body time to adjust. It can be difficult and frustrating to make abrupt and significant changes to one's eating habits. Ensure you are meeting your nutrient needs while gradually introducing new meals and eliminating others.

Keep in mind that no one diet works for everyone. Everybody has different nutritional requirements, tastes, and objectives. Finding a sustainable strategy that promotes your general health and is compatible with your particular situation is essential when choosing the proper food diet. You can make an informed choice and start along the path of healthy eating by taking into account the aforementioned considerations and, if necessary, consulting a specialist.

CHAPTER 4.

IMPLEMENTING A FOOD DIET.

Putting a food diet into practice entails making deliberate decisions regarding the kinds and amounts of food you eat in order to attain particular health or lifestyle goals. When putting a food plan into practice, keep the following points in mind:

Set your objectives: Establish your goals for implementing a food plan in detail. Are you trying to follow a particular eating plan (vegetarian, vegan, ketogenic, etc.) or are you hoping to lose weight, build muscle, or enhance your general health?

Consult a healthcare professional: Before beginning a new food plan, it is usually a good idea to speak with a healthcare provider or a qualified dietitian. Based on your particular requirements, medical background, and any underlying issues, they can offer tailored advice.

Learn about macronutrients: Carbohydrates, proteins, and lipids are examples of macronutrients. A balanced diet is necessary for good health because each of these macronutrients has a crucial function in the body. You can plan your meals more effectively if you are aware of the recommended intake and sources of each macronutrient.

Think about portion control: It's crucial to do so even when eating nutritious foods. Portion control is important to prevent overeating. You can estimate the proper portions with the aid of tools like measuring cups, food scales, and visual cues.

Emphasize full, nutritious foods: Give entire, unprocessed foods that are nutrient-rich a priority. Fruits, vegetables, whole grains, lean meats, and healthy fats are a few of these. These foods supply necessary fiber, antioxidants, vitamins, and minerals.

Proper hydration is essential for good health in general. Make an effort to get enough water throughout the day. The suggested intake varies according to the environment, level of physical activity, and personal demands.

Planning and preparing meals in advance will help you maintain a balanced and wholesome diet. This can assist you in avoiding impulsive eating selections and helping you make better choices. Furthermore, cooking your food gives you control over the ingredients and cooking techniques.

Practice mindful eating by being aware of your body's signals of hunger and fullness. To prevent overeating, take your time eating, appreciate the flavors, and pay attention to your body's cues.

Flexibility and adaptation: Keep in mind that no one diet is right for everyone. It's crucial to choose a strategy that complements your way of life, tastes, and medical needs. Be flexible when making changes, and if necessary, try out other food regimens.

Monitoring your progress can help you stay inspired and make any necessary corrections along the road. This can involve keeping an eye on things like weight, physical measurements, energy levels, and general health.

Consistency and sustainability: Adopting a food diet works best when it transforms into a permanent lifestyle shift as opposed to a quick fix. To achieve and sustain your targeted goals, consistency, and long-term dedication are essential.

Always seek expert advice from a trained dietician or healthcare provider to receive recommendations that are tailored to your specific requirements and circumstances.

CHAPTER 5.

COMMON CHALLENGES IN FOOD DIET.

Many people find starting a food diet to be a difficult task. Despite the fact that specific difficulties can differ based on the type of food and an individual's unique situation, there are several typical difficulties that people frequently encounter. Following a food diet can be difficult for the reasons listed below.

Dealing with cravings and hunger is one of the most frequent problems with diets that involve eating. Cravings for comfortable, frequently less healthful foods are common when changing to a new eating routine or cutting calories. Additionally, it could take some time for the body to acclimate to smaller portions, which could result in hunger.

Participating in social activities and gatherings can be difficult for people on a food diet because of social pressures and temptations. There may be pressure to indulge in unhealthy meals from friends and family members who don't fully understand or support the dietary limitations. When confronted with a range of mouthwatering delicacies that are off-limits at events or restaurants, temptations may strike.

Emotional Eating: Emotional eating can make it extremely difficult to keep up a healthy diet. Comfort foods, which are frequently heavy in calories and lacking in nutrition, can be desired as a result of stress, boredom, melancholy, or other emotions. Overcoming this difficulty requires managing emotional triggers and developing other coping strategies.

Lack of Time and Convenience: It might be challenging to maintain a diet due to a busy schedule and a lack of time. In comparison to choosing fast, processed foods, preparing healthy meals frequently takes more time and effort. This difficulty can be overcome by finding methods to organize food preparation, meal planning, and cooking.

Monotony and Limited Food Options: Some diets may have restrictions on the kind of meals that are permitted, which could result in a limited menu and monotony. Eating the same things regularly might get monotonous and make it difficult to maintain a diet over time. To overcome this obstacle, try out new recipes, play around with different ingredients, and include a wide variety of wholesome foods.

Nutritional Imbalance: Adopting particular dietary regimens without the right instruction or comprehension may result in nutritional imbalances. Deficits in vital nutrients, vitamins, and minerals can occur on restrictive diets that cut out entire food groups. Any diet should be well-balanced and have all the elements required for good health, therefore it's crucial to make sure of that.

Lack of Support and Accountability: Trying a food plan on your own can make it tough to stay motivated and hold yourself accountable. Without assistance from friends, family, or a community, it's simpler to become distracted and fall back on old routines. Overcoming this difficulty can be facilitated by establishing a support network, participating in online forums, or consulting a dietitian or nutritionist.

Weight Reduction Plateaus and Slow Progress: People on a food diet may become discouraged when they experience weight reduction plateaus or slow progress. Following initial success, weight reduction may slow down and the body's metabolism may adjust, making future advancement difficult. A plateau can be broken with dedication, patience, and adopting exercise or other lifestyle adjustments.

Lack of Education and Guidance: Beginning a diet without the right information and support can be difficult. People may find it difficult to make wise decisions if they don't grasp the nutritional requirements and how to design a balanced diet. A safe and efficient strategy can be ensured by consulting a licensed dietician or healthcare expert.

Unrealistic Expectations: Having unattainable expectations might make you angry and disappointed. It might be harmful to one's general well-being to lose weight quickly or to strive for an unrealistic body image. The secret to overcoming this difficulty is to put your attention on your long-term health, slow growth, and enduring habits.

The journey for a healthy life.

It's crucial to keep in mind that each person's experience with food diets might be unique, and these issues can differ in severity and importance. The likelihood of success can be considerably increased by developing individualized plans, getting expert advice, and having a flexible mindset.

CHAPTER 6.

CONCLUSION AND FINAL THOUGHTS ON FOOD DIET.

In conclusion, it is impossible to emphasize the effect that our diet has on how we feel in general. For preserving good health and preventing numerous chronic diseases, a well-balanced and nourishing diet is crucial. We have changed the way we eat over time, and with so many options available now, it is more crucial than ever to choose our food carefully.

We can provide our bodies with the nutrition they need to function well by consuming a balanced, varied diet. In order to do this, we must include a mix of fruits, vegetables, whole grains, lean meats, and healthy fats in our meals. Additionally, it requires controlling the use of processed foods, added sweets, and harmful fats.

Individual factors, such as age, activity level, and any existing medical issues, must be taken into account because nutritional needs might differ from person to person. In order to guarantee that dietary decisions are in line with particular needs and objectives, consulting with healthcare specialists such as registered dietitians can offer individualized counsel.

Developing a healthy connection with food is also essential. Avoiding rigid diets and categorizing foods as "good" or "bad" can help to prevent harmful eating habits and encourage a healthy mindset. A more sustainable and satisfying eating experience can be attained by adopting a flexible strategy that allows for splurging occasionally or honoring ethnic traditions.

Beyond our personal health, our food choices have an impact. Our food choices ought to make ethical and sustainable issues into account. Reducing food waste, adopting organic and ethically sourced ingredients, and promoting local farmers are all crucial steps in developing a more environmentally and socially responsible food system.

To sum up, our diet is more than just a source of nutrition; it is an essential part of our entire well-being and has a significant impact on our health, the environment, and society at large. We may nourish our bodies, safeguard the environment, and contribute to a healthy future for present generations by putting an emphasis on a balanced diet, personalized choices, and conscious consumerism.

SUMMARY OF KEY POINTS ON FOOD DIET.

Diets are a crucial part of preserving good health and well-being. Among the most crucial factors are:

Various nutrient-dense foods, such as fruits, vegetables, whole grains, lean meats, and healthy fats, should be included in a healthy diet.

Making nutritional decisions should take into account a person's dietary requirements, lifestyle considerations, and cultural influences.

Guidance and assistance can be obtained by speaking with a qualified dietician or healthcare practitioner.
By eating a nutritious diet, one can increase their energy levels, manage their chronic medical issues, and lower their risk of contracting chronic illnesses.

Making informed decisions about food selections and dietary patterns can be facilitated by educating oneself on the fundamentals of nutrition and dietary requirements, obtaining reliable sources of information, and experimenting with different foods and dishes.

A holistic approach can help support lifetime health and vigor, and the advantages of a good diet are well worth the effort.

LONG TERM BENEFITS OF FOOD DIET.

The long-term advantages of maintaining a good diet for wellness and general health are numerous. These advantages include:

Reduced chance of developing chronic diseases: A balanced diet can lower your risk of getting conditions like heart disease, type 2 diabetes, and some types of cancer. This is due to the fact that a diet full of fruits, vegetables, whole grains, and lean meats offers crucial nutrients and antioxidants that support a strong immune system and normal cellular activity.

Better control of weight: A healthy food diet can help you control your weight by encouraging feelings of fullness and lowering your chance of overeating. Additionally, it can lessen the risk of obesity and related medical problems.

Increased energy: A good diet can provide you constant energy throughout the day, preventing drops in blood sugar and lessening symptoms of exhaustion.

An improved diet that includes healthy foods can help to enhance the brain's health and cognitive performance. Omega-3 fatty acids are included in a number of foods, including nuts and fatty fish, and they support the health of the brain.

Improved mood: Eating healthily can also boost your mood and lower your risk of sadness and anxiety. This is due to the role that some minerals, like magnesium and the B vitamins, play in mood regulation.

Overall, it is impossible to emphasize the advantages of a diet high in healthful foods. People can enhance their long-term health and well-being by including a variety of nutrient-dense foods in their diets and implementing sustainable dietary modifications.

TIPS FOR SUCCESS IN A FOOD DIET.

It can be difficult to switch to a healthy diet, but the following advice will help boost your chances of success:

Create attainable, concrete, quantifiable, and time-bound goals as a starting point. You may monitor your development and maintain motivation in this way.

Make adjustments gradually: Rather than attempting to completely revamp your diet all at once, it's crucial to make changes to your diet gradually. This can make it easier and more sustainable to switch to a healthy diet.

Plan and prepare meals in advance to make sure there are always nutritious options accessible. Lack of time or options can also lessen the possibility that bad meal choices will be made.

Seek assistance: To keep yourself on track and motivated, ask for help from family and friends or think about joining a support group.

Try new foods: Trying new foods and recipes helps keep your diet interesting.

Keep hydrated: Throughout the day, drinking plenty of water might help you feel full and lower your risk of overeating.

Follow your progress: Monitoring your progress helps keep you inspired and shows you where you might need to make dietary changes.

People can successfully switch to a healthy food diet and take advantage of all its advantages by putting these suggestions into practice and developing a positive outlook. entertaining and fascinating.

Thank you for reading, do have a wonderful and healthy diet that will maintain your body system and keep you fit for the rest of your life. If you find this book worthy, don't forget to let others know about it. Do have a happy reading and a successful diet plan.